FITNESS
The Answer Book

Books in This Series

Fitness: The Answer Book by Cecil B. Murphey

Flab: The Answer Book by Jim Krafft, M.D.

Headaches: The Answer Book by Joan Miller, Ph.D.

Heart Attacks: The Answer Book by Daniel J. MacNeil, M.D., and Larry Losoncy, Ph.D.

Junk Food: The Answer Book by Virginia and Norman Rohrer

Vitamins: The Answer Book by Virginia and Norman Rohrer

FITNESS
The Answer Book

Cecil B. Murphey

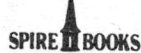

Fleming H. Revell Company
Old Tappan, New Jersey

ISBN: 0-8007-8466-9

A Spire Book
Copyright © 1983 Fleming H. Revell Company
All rights reserved
Printed in the United States of America

Before starting any fitness program, a medical doctor should be consulted.

CONTENTS

Introduction 9
1 *Be a Better You!* 13
2 *What's the Good of It?* 15
3 *In Shape? Who, Me?* 21
4 *The Shape-Up Craze* 25
5 *The Experts Speak* 29
6 *Getting Psyched Up* 31
7 *Four Problems* 37
8 *To Diet, to Diet* 39
9 *Which Body Type Are You?* 43
10 *How Dense Are You?* 49
11 *Isometric, Isotonic, and Those Other Strange Words* 51
12 *Toes in the Water* 53
13 *Before You Do Your First Exercise* 57
14 *A Word About Breathing* 61
15 *Shape-Up Exercises* 63
16 *Don't-Just-Sit-There Exercises* 67
17 *Cheating Exercises* 71
18 *Stick With It* 79
19 *To Sleep . . .* 83
20 *An Added Bonus: Sharper Minds!* 85
21 *Results?* 87
22 *Miscellaneous Fitness Tips* 89
23 *If You've Got the Money . . .* 91
24 *Finally . . .* 93
For Further Reading 94

INTRODUCTION

There's an old story in medicine about the doctor who wearied of treating typhoid patients and put a lock on the source of the epidemic, the town pump. The best doctors always have an eye out for ways of preventing illness—while working industriously on the cure.

The great advances of modern medicine have made most of us live longer, thereby uncovering such disorders as coronary artery disease, stroke, and senility. These are now some of the most challenging frontiers of medical research and care. The sources of these disorders are many, but the "town pump" we can get a hand on lies in the life-style of the patient. Dealing with this has proved harder than coping with typhoid bacillus!

Selling patients on changing their daily habits, on the diet, exercise, and moderation that are the "wonder drugs" of the eighties requires expert salesmanship—something doctors are not very good at. We are frustrated by inertia, boredom, and the skepticism most reasonable people have of the quickie, crash programs flooding the book market today.

Books like this one of Cec Murphey's are just what the doctor ordered. His plain common sense, his enthusiasm, and his sensitivity to the pitfalls that foil so many plans, make this the kind of prescription I would like to keep on the corner of my desk to hand out to those who need a nudge to get started. It is a safe way to start and a sane way to get fit.

The best testimonial I have for the effectiveness of this book is what has happened to Cec himself. I have known him during the entire time of his transformation from flab to fitness and know that this "doctor" has taken his own medicine.

That's not a bad idea. That bulge sticking out below my belt isn't the tailor's padding! Maybe, the first of next week, I'll start . . .

No, I'll start—let's *both* start—*today!*

C. MARKHAM BERRY, M.D.

FITNESS
The Answer Book

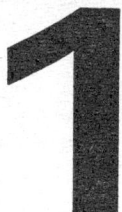

Be a Better You!

Remember when you wore a size eight and you prided yourself on your tiny waistline?

Remember when Mom said you had a bottomless pit for a stomach, because you ate constantly but didn't gain weight? When older folks kept trying to fatten you up?

Do you sigh, recalling those bygone days, silently wishing you could be thin, healthy looking, and in shape once again?

You can be.

Would you like to run up a flight of stairs or chase the kids across the yard and not pant for breath? How would you like to get back into those clothes you wore in high school?

You can do it.

How would you feel if someone who hadn't seen you for ten years said, "Why, I hardly recognized you. You look so young—and in such good shape"?

It can happen to you!

How would you like to feel good—really good—about yourself? Wouldn't it be great not to wear your clothes loose to cover blobs of fat? Wouldn't you like to peek at your reflection in store windows, smile, and think, *I look great?*

You can do it.

That's the purpose of this book—to help you become a better you.

You can be just that—healthier
> happier
>> more self-confident
>>> and more energetic.

I don't have a magic potion or offer a surefire money-back guarantee that you'll end up like a pro athlete.

Here's what I can offer you—hope
> help
>> awareness of the possibilities for a better you.

This can happen, even if you're—badly out of shape
> sixty pounds overweight
>> controlled by a never-quitting appetite
>>> have no willpower.

You can be a better you
> without expensive equipment
>> without hours of daily exercise
>>> without stringent diets of boring meals and a list of no-no foods.

Do you want to get into shape?
> Do you want to be the best YOU possible?
>> Want to look your best
>>> feel your best
>>>> and have others see you at your best?

Do you want to be able to say,
> "Thanks, God, for me"?

This may be the book you've been waiting to read.

2

What's the Good of It?

"Why should I get myself into shape?" Edna asked. "I know I'm a little overweight," she admitted. Her dresses bulged in the wrong places, and she no longer possessed the energy level she had at age twenty. She took another potato chip, covered it with a creamy dip, and said, "What's so good about getting into shape?"

I told her about my own shape-up program. I added that with regular exercise and a sensible diet, life had changed drastically for me.

"In what way?" she asked.

"I feel good about myself—really good."

"Through exercise and diet?"

"Absolutely," I said.

I explained that I hadn't started a shape-up program for that reason, "but it's one of the by-products of getting into shape."

"Very nice," she said and reached for another chip, "but I'm not much into all that sweating and ten hours a week of exercise and strict diets."

"Did I say anything about that?"

"No, but . . ."

"Getting into shape doesn't *have* to make you feel like a

zombie for six months. In fact, it can be fun. At least, it was for me."

I remembered how intimidated those brawny types had made me feel—broad shoulders, trim waist, and symmetrical biceps. I'd suck in my gut, hoping people wouldn't compare us.

"You're not a muscleman," Edna said, "but you're trim."

"And I feel great!"

"You look it."

"It's affected my whole life," I added. "Not only did I get my body shaped up, but it's affected my outlook on life, my energy level. Why, people frequently think I'm at least ten years younger than I am."

Edna pushed the potato chips away and plied me with questions, especially when I told her that I never exercised until I was over forty.

As I explained to Edna, when our bodies are in the kind of shape God created them to be in, we not only have a more efficient system with fewer aches and minor physical problems, but we enjoy life more.

We talked for almost an hour, and Edna gave me every excuse she could think of for not shaping up. She finally said, "I'm not disciplined enough, I guess."

"You need self-discipline, of course," I said, "but it's more a matter of decision. Once you decide you want to get into shape—decide seriously enough to take action—you've halfway won the battle."

I pointed out that, as one of my writer friends says, "The fat is in your head." Get your head thinking right, and you'll lose the bulges.

"And, Edna, you might look ten years younger—you'll certainly *feel* younger."

"Really?"

"Right. Some experts insist that shaping up retards aging. The evidence isn't all in, but we do know this much: Even if you haven't set the clock back, you look younger because you're in shape. You also enjoy life more because you feel better."

Eventually Edna, too, became an avid devotee of physical fitness.

Think about it. I know I'm in the best shape I can be for my age and my general build.

Don't take my word for it. Ask others who have shaped up. They'll give you wonderful physical reports—

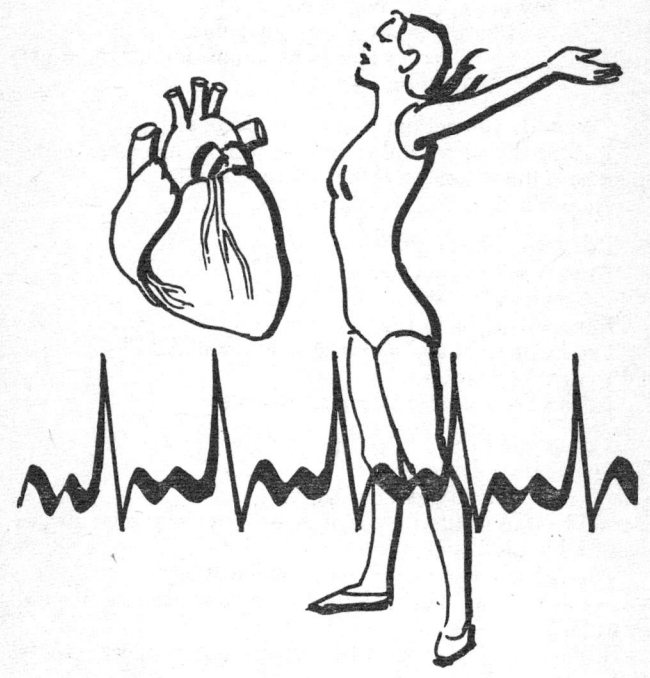

Steadier heart rhythm can be a benefit of a fitness program.

lowered blood pressure
    less anxiety
        steadier heart rhythm
            healthier-looking skin
                lower cholesterol levels.

Here's what Edna said eight months later:

    "My posture has improved.
        I have less stiffness in my joints.
            I don't suffer from chronic fatigue the way I used to."

"What do you get out of physical exercise?"

I asked this of several friends as well as members of the American Fitness Center, in Jonesboro, Georgia.

Here is a sampling of their replies:

- "I've got more energy."
- "Greater self-esteem."
- "I'm more optimistic about life."
- "I'm not as tense as I used to be."
- "I've lost weight and inches around my middle."
- "I fall asleep quicker."
- "I don't need as much sleep as I used to."

Consistent
    and regular exercise
        makes these changes!

Many of us adults are out of shape. But we haven't always been flabby, tired, and achy.

Think back. Remember your childhood days.

As children we didn't need to be urged to exercise. We did it naturally.

Unfortunately, we tend to decrease our physical activity after the age of twenty-five.

Then the results of soft living hit us:

- Flab develops.
- Muscle tone decreases and muscles atrophy.
- This causes more flab.
- The muscle tone decreases . . .

and the cycle goes on.

Most people not only decrease or stop their exercise at twenty-five, they also fail to cut down on their food intake—

What's the Good of It?

eating as much at forty as they did twenty years earlier, when they were more physically active.

Once we reach thirty, we need fewer calories every year!
That's not all...

Instead of continued physical activity and lower caloric intake, we stretch out on a comfortable sofa. We put only the same small group of muscles through repetitive patterns of action. Day after day, year after year.

Yet...
    we have more than 600 muscles and 200 bones.

Putting it into practical terms, to stay firm, strong, and flexible:

We   need   exercise.

> Exercise strengthens while
> inactivity wastes.
>   HIPPOCRATES

3

In Shape? Who, Me?

Although this is the second book I've written on physical fitness, I sometimes marvel that of all subjects, I'm writing on this one.

With the exception of bowling, I never excelled in sports. That's not quite right—I wasn't good at sports. Too short for basketball, too small for football, and when it came to soccer, I lacked the required coordination. I couldn't bat or catch a fly ball any better than Charlie Brown.

And now, years later, I'm involved and writing in the area of physical fitness. I'm an avid jogger (and have been since 1977), chalking up more than thirty miles a week. I'm an average swimmer. I don't lift weights, run marathons, or play team sports; but I am in good physical shape.

As I near the half-century mark of life and look critically at myself, I can say, "Yep, I'm in excellent physical shape for my age."

But it wasn't always so.

Eight years ago I got serious about physical well-being and gradually moved into a regimen that put me into good shape.

Today, besides my running, I do a few calisthenics. I've radically changed my eating style. My doctor tells me my heart ought to keep me going until I'm at least one hundred. I'm trim and weigh less than I did in high school.

Most of all, I feel good about myself. I like the shape I'm in, and it gives me positive feelings about myself.

I've written all this at the beginning of the book because I have gotten myself into shape—and I'm not a college athlete. I'll never look like a football player (I'm built thin and wiry). *But I am in shape.*

I became conscious of how much I'd changed when I returned to my hometown last summer for a high school reunion. After an interval of nearly thirty years, I saw my fellow classmates again.

Jay stood just inside the door. As a senior, he had bulging muscles, which he flexed from time to time. He knocked many opponents flat as he plowed across the football field.

"Is that you, Jay?" I asked uncertainly.

"Sure is," he said, "guess I've gotten a little bald since you saw me last."

"Yes, you have," I said and shook hands. His once-bulging muscles looked more like a prolapsed stomach and two sagging chins.

Ellie, the tennis champ and top female track star sat during the entire evening—she now weighed nearly 300 pounds and complained of emphysema, diabetes, and high blood pressure.

But two of us gained attention. Lila had always been chubby. She was the type to whom people remarked, "But you have such a pretty face." Now Lila had a pretty body to match.

No one recognized me. When I introduced myself, one classmate said, "But—but you've gotten so skinny."

What music to the ears of someone who had lost thirty pounds and tightened his waistline four inches! My classmate, on the other hand, had added a hundred pounds to his own frame.

I haven't always been in good shape. In 1970 I had my first attack of ulcers and wound up in the hospital. My doctor warned me then about high blood pressure.

I knew I was overweight, but undernourished, and out of shape. I had a sloppy waistline that I tried to hide by wearing a suit jacket—always unbuttoned.

Then, after a second trip to the hospital and three less-serious ulcer attacks, I decided to do something about myself.

I read everything I could about nutrition and physical fit-

In Shape? Who, Me?

ness. I asked questions. Through trial and error (a lot of errors!) I developed a regimen that put me into good shape.

My weight has remained constant for the past six years. I need no medication, other than occasional antihistamine for sinus problems, and still maintain a high energy level.

Frankly, I feel better today than I did when I was thirty!

And in this book I'd like to share with you what I've learned about physical well-being.

I'm not writing for those who want to model for Mr. America ads or enter beauty contests.

I'm writing this book for the rest of us—the ordinary people who don't like bulging hips and thighs, who feel embarrassed about the five inches hanging over our belt buckles and want to do something about it.

You can get into shape.

It's not easy. It's discipline

                commitment

                        time . . . but you can do it.

I did it!
You can, too!

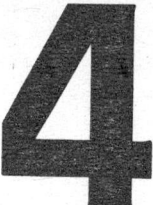

The Shape-Up Craze

Did you know that *today*—or any day—more than 70 million Americans will practice some form of physical exercise? That's half our adult population. And yet, according to the November 2, 1981 issue of *Time* magazine, only about one-fourth of the population exercised regularly in 1961.

Jogging, for instance, has been growing in popularity for more than a decade. The Peachtree Road race, run annually in Atlanta on July 4, has had to *limit* entrants to the first 25,000. The Boston Marathon, because of its increased popularity, now is limited to those who can meet certain standards of performance.

Football players of the Los Angeles Rams attended jazzercise classes twice weekly in the spring of 1982 in an attempt to stay in shape and keep limber during their off-season.

The Serious Athletes
Statistics indicate that Americans have become serious about physical fitness. Consider these figures as estimated by experts in the field. America now has:

- More than 20 million runners
- 6 million (mostly women) jazzercisers, dancercisers, or aerobic dancers

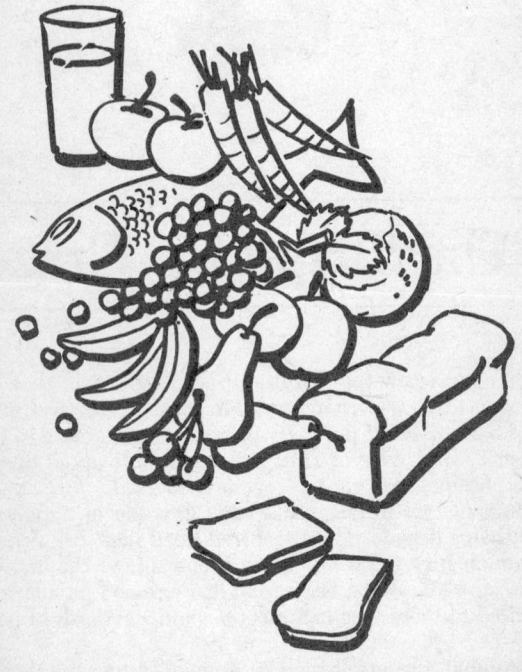

Fitness-conscious Americans are choosing a more nutritious diet.

The Shape-Up Craze

- 13 million biceps builders
- 20 million on a diet right now.

We're also listening to warnings about too much sugar
> too much salt
>> the addition of preservatives and
>>> additives to our food
>>>> and we're learning to eat balanced meals.

We now read package labels in the supermarket

> as we search for artificial ingredients
> and hidden poisons, and
>> we love the word *natural*.

Books such as James Fixx's *The Complete Book of Running* and *Jane Brody's Nutrition Book*

> have hit
>> and stayed
>>> on the best-seller lists for months.

Fitness-conscious Americans can recite information
> about vitamins and minerals
>> and are moving toward more simplified meals
>>> avoiding heavy starches
>>>> rich desserts
>>>>> and are moderating in the amount of red meat, and whole milk products we use.

Even the fast-food chains now offer salad bars,
> and we're eating more green and yellow vegetables
>> whole grains
>>> and fruits.

We have rediscovered
> miller's bran (the residue from the production of white flour)
>> which not only aids in bowel regulation but possibly is beneficial in preventing diverticulitis and cancer of the colon.

5

The Experts Speak

Recognizing the fitness boom in our country, a question-and-answer column in *Better Living* (June, 1982) asked, "What do you do to keep in shape?"

Top cardiologists answered the question, each urging people to get involved in a personal fitness program. All but one spoke of his own fitness program (and most of them listed jogging).

One expert pleaded for people to stay in motion with what he called nonstructured exercises, such as standing instead of sitting, moving around frequently, and taking stairs instead of elevators.

Nicholas Kounovsky, author of *The Joy of Feeling Fit*, and vocal exponent of physical fitness, has served as consultant to national and international organizations, foundations, and publications. He says, "Fitness makes for joy in living."

Eleanor Metheny writes in *Connotations of Movement in Sport and Dance*:

> We [women] play tennis for the same reason that men paint pictures, sing, play musical instruments, devise and solve algebraic equations, and fly aeroplanes ... because it satisfies our human need to use our human abilities, to experience ourselves as

significant, creative, and, therefore, personalized beings in an impersonal world.

Kathryn Lance, author of several books on fitness, including *Running for Health and Beauty* and *Getting Strong*, said she was a 120-pound weakling. After getting into a fitness program that included weightlifting, she felt much stronger after only twelve weeks. "I had also improved my figure and general well-being. Best of all, I was able to maintain my new level of strength by exercising only once or twice a week. The exercises, which had been difficult at first, became easier and more pleasant week by week."

Katherine Switzer, the first woman to run in the Boston Marathon, said in an interview, "Sports are as natural—and as good—for women as they are for men."

6

Getting Psyched Up

Before I try to get you psyched up, I want to tell you how I psyched up myself.

"You need to exercise," I told my flabby reflection in the mirror.

My reflection agreed.

Unfortunately, I made one tactical error. I said, "I'll start a serious program next week."

Within a week my commitment to physical shaping up had died like hundreds of other ideas for self-improvement.

Two years later, I said, "I'll run—starting today." *And* I followed through.

First, I measured one mile with the car—half a mile out and half a mile back.

Then, in sloppy clothes and walking shoes (not knowing much about running shoes) I started out.

I burst into full speed—and for at least ten seconds I felt great. I didn't even reach a quarter of a mile before I stopped, fell to the ground and panted. Minutes later, I huffed as I walked back home.

During the following year I would start a shape-up program and stay with it for a couple of weeks; then I'd miss a day.

Once I started to miss exercise days, I was ready to quit again.
Then, tired of my flab,
> scared of my soaring blood pressure
> concerned because of my lack of energy

I prayed.
> "God, I'm going to shape up. I'll do everything I can.
> Help me stick with it. Don't let me give up."

That was eight years ago. I'm still at it.

It happened like this: Howard, a thirty-five-year-old and the victim of a heart attack, worked out three times a week at a health spa.

He invited me to go with him. I joined the first day.

"I want a program to get me into shape and tone up my muscles," I told an instructor at the spa.

The instructor gave me a list of exercises that took about twenty minutes. (Most of these exercises could have been done at home without any special equipment.)

That's how I got started.

Others have psyched themselves up differently.

Wilma and three friends get together five mornings a week for a lengthy walk. They've been doing it for three years.

Two businessmen go into the equipment room at lunch and do calisthenics together for ten minutes each workday.

My daughter Cecile got into running by reading books and magazines on the subject.

A friend said, "Everyone in my neighborhood started trimming down and shaping up. Whenever we had neighborhood gatherings, fitness became the central topic of conversation. I started exercising and joined a raquetball club so that I could feel part of our community again."

If you're not already involved in a shape-up program, do something to get yourself enthused.
> Such as . . .

Read books on health.
> Subscribe to fitness magazines.
>> Ask friends.
>>> Check on programs and courses on getting into shape offered by recreation centers
>>> the "Y"
>>> your local college
>>> the office or factory where you work.

Getting Psyched Up

We all notice people who are in good physical shape, often staring in envy not only at their body contours
> but their graceful walk
>> their sense of well-being
>>> their look of self-assurance.

Do you know someone like that?
> She may be a co-worker
>> someone who attends the same church you do
>>> maybe a neighbor.

Select such a person and start a conversation:
> "You look as though you're in great shape,"
>> you say. "How do you do it?"

Most people who walked the flabby road, and left it by shaping up, become wildly enthusiastic when asked such a question. They'll often give you all kinds of hints. (They might even agree to help you get started.)

Try this:

> Each morning, stand naked in front of your mirror.
> Stare at yourself.
> Say aloud,
>> "God made this body.
>> I'm responsible for taking care of it
>> and keeping it in shape."

Here's another tip.

> Think of yourself as a house owned by someone else, in which you're the tenant.

"You're responsible for doing repairs, cutting the grass, and whatever needs doing, but you pay no rent," the owner says.

How would the owner respond to seeing the yard overgrown with weeds, garbage on the back steps, and windows broken?

Apply that idea to yourself. "What can I do to this body to show God I want to take care of it?"

Read everything you can about physical fitness *and* disease. Learn about hypertension, emphysema and other respiratory ailments, heart disease, diabetes. This is not to frighten but to inform—*and*
> as a reinforcement to

get your body into shape.

Join a biking club or one devoted to bikers and joggers. In most metropolitan areas, the local newspaper lists weekly sports activities. Take up a sport—but make sure it's one that requires constant motion. Racquetball, running, walking, and swimming have good overall benefits. Tennis requires a lot of movement for poor players. (The better you get, the less you move!) What about an aerobic-dancing class? Take up clogging or square dancing.

Many of the above involve participating with others. For some people, that's the only way to get psyched up to begin. Most important,

SET A GOAL FOR YOURSELF.

Make it a realistic one.

For instance, it may be as simple as, "In three months I will walk two full miles, four times a week."

Write out your goal.

Display your goal on the refrigerator.

> Tape it to your mirror.
>
> Put a copy on the dashboard of your car.
>
> Why not take one copy to work? Tape it just inside a drawer you open several times a day.

Stop right now. Write down your goal:

_____

_____

_____

Find ways to remind yourself of this goal.

Tell your friends. Urge them to ask you each week for a progress report.

My wife found that putting up slogans and cartoons in the kitchen helped her stay away from excess food and reminded her of her goal to get into shape.

GOD DOESN'T WANT ME
   TO BE FAT.

                             TASTE MAKES WAIST

A friend has this over her sink.

   DON'T BE A HUMAN
     GARBAGE CAN

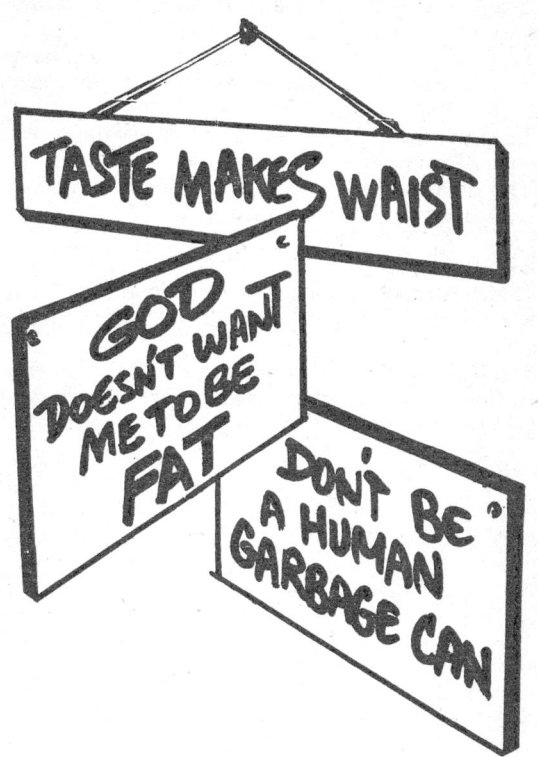

*Putting up signs can remind
us to stick to our goal of shaping up.*

Next to the scales, at a local health spa, they have an enlarged colored photo of a glob of fat with the caption:
> This is what five pounds of extra fat
> looks like.

Try *imaging*.

Imaging, a technique that has come into wide use in the last decade, works like this.

Look at yourself frequently in a mirror or a glass window. In your mind, however, envision yourself the way you'd *like* to be.

Keep this image before you daily—every time you catch a reflection of yourself.

This constant input of positive self-imaging can help motivate you to act out your imaging.

Try prayer.

God cares about you because he created you. Ask his help in your proposed program. Ask him to help you discipline yourself.

> P.S., Also, forgive yourself in those instances when you neglect your exercise program for a few days or blow your diet.

7

Four Problems

Since I've become addicted to fitness, I talk to people about shaping up. I've heard dozens of excuses, reasons, and problems.

The four problem areas most commonly mentioned are:

1. *"I don't have time."*

Wrong. We have time for what we believe is important. If concern for our health and general well-being become important to us, we will find time. We all do the things we consider important. As long as we complain, "I don't have time," we're actually saying, "Fitness isn't that important."

2. *"I don't have the energy."*

We hear people say, "When I get home from work, I'm so tired, I just want to collapse."

Or, "By the time I get the kids to bed, I'm too worn out for anything physical."

That's the time to get into shape. If you were in good shape, you wouldn't be that tired out.

Further, the tiredness probably has not come from physical activity *but from the lack of it.*

3. *"Women who train look like amazons and lose their femininity."*

Actually, it's the opposite. Women who lift weights, for example, develop *firm* muscles, but because of their thicker subcutaneous layer of fat, they don't bulge the way men do.

More important, the female body retains its contours. Muscular development of the chest improves the bust line. The thighs and hips, the real trouble spots, are s-l-i-m-m-e-d by exercise.

4. *"But I ..."*

This covers any other problems you have that prevent your getting into shape.

But if you want to *look* your best
> *feel* your best
> have more energy
> and retard aging,

you'll realize that instead of problems, you have a great opportunity. You can even say, "I'm going to get into shape, starting today."

8

To Diet, to Diet

For most people, getting in shape means that horrid word:
diet.

Whether they feel the need to round off an inch at the hips, and two at the waist, or for an overall slimming program, they continue to face the starkness of the word.

A friend recently said, "Is it an accident that the word *die* is there? When I try to lose pounds, I feel as though that's what I'm going to do—die!"

To diet . . . to diet . . .

But before thinking about specific diets, let's look at food.

Food—we all need it. Among other reasons, because it supplies our energy.

Experts long ago classified four basic food groups to help us in getting a well-balanced diet every day:

milk and dairy products

    meat and other high-protein foods such as fish and eggs

        fruits and vegetables

            grains (as in bread) and cereals

All diets revolve around these four food groups, restricting some, forbidding others, insisting on a few, and suggesting additional portions.

Body weight follows a simple rule. When we eat more food than we need to meet the demands of our body, we store the excess in our body as fat. And we gain weight.

If we eat less than our body demands, we take energy from those fat deposits and burn them up. We lose weight.

Before you rush out to try a newly published diet, here are a few things to bear in mind:

Jane Brody, in *Jane Brody's Nutrition Book,* emphasizes that no one diet fits everyone's problem. We're all different with different needs. She also acknowledges that some people need a "higher authority" to tell them

>> what to avoid
>> and what to eat.

For such people,
> a structured diet may be the answer.

But no matter what diet you choose, bear in mind these three things:

1. There's no shortcut to thinness.
2. You probably took years to put on your excess weight. Be willing to take a year to get it back off, especially if you're 20 percent, or more, overweight.
3. The real answer for keeping off pounds isn't a perpetual diet, but devising a new life-style—
> a life-style of eating
>> *and* exercising that keeps you healthy
>>> provides nutritionally balanced meals
>>> doesn't deprive you of the pleasures of food.

Current, popular diets for weight reduction include:

1. The high protein, low-carbohydrate diets. Whether it's Dr. Atkins' Diet Revolution or Dr. Stillman's Quick Weight Loss Diet, they all emphasize protein and/or fat. This heavy use of fat is risky because of the resulting high intake of cholesterol and saturated fats. Nutritionists cited in *Rating the Diets* by Theodore Berland and the editors of *Consumer Guide* have condemned these diets as dangerous.

According to *Time* magazine (November 2, 1981), the two diets with the poorest medical marks are the Atkins Diet and the Beverly Hills Diet (which is discussed below.)

2. The Woman Doctor's Diet for Women, originated by Barbara Edelstein, comes out of her own practice. Dr. Edelstein is a physician specializing in overweight, and she contends that women lose weight differently, and more slowly, than men. This fact hasn't been taken into account by most leading diets.

To Diet, to Diet

She provides a high-protein, low-carbohydrate diet because she believes that women, especially the overweight, handle protein more efficiently than carbohydrates.

Arguments against high-protein, low-carbohydrate diets apply here. The recommended fat intake, after the first two weeks, reaches 50 percent, which nutritionists consider too high to be healthy.

3. *The Pritikin Diet*, while high in complex carbohydrates such as whole grains, fruits, and vegetables, is low in fat and protein. Designed originally for people with heart disease, this diet also provides for high-bulk foods and snacking between meals. Pritikin theorizes that the body functions best when food is eaten more frequently.

Experts say that the Pritikin Diet takes a basically sound idea and carries it to an extreme. He advocates an austere (some call it boring), difficult-to-follow menu. Myron Winick, of the Institute of Human Nutrition at Columbia University, is quoted in *Time* (November 2, 1981) as saying, "If you follow it, you almost can't eat in a restaurant."

4. *The Beverly Hills Diet*, created by Judy Mazel, allows nothing but fruit for the first week. You may have as much as you want, provided one fruit is digested before you eat another.

Mazel's theory is that different enzymes digest different kinds of foods. The secret is not to mix types of food but to let enzymes work, otherwise you inhibit digestion and the food turns to fat.

After the second week, you eat vegetables and bread, and by the third week, lobster. But the eat-them-separately theory still holds.

The *Journal of the American Medical Association* has called the diet hazardous to health. Leading nutritionists oppose this protein-deficient diet, citing also the lack of calcium, iron, thiamin, niacin, and riboflavin.

5. *The Weight Watchers Diet*, developed by Jean Nidetch to cure her own weight problems, has been revised several times. The present diet offers three variations (full choice, 1,200 calories daily; limited choice, 1,100; and no choice, 1,050).

The program, never published in book form, is available only to members of Weight Watchers who pay a registration fee and weekly fee for classes. The diet plan provides for support from the group, behavior modification, and exercise. Of all the leading diets in the past decade, this is the one that has received high marks from most experts as being sensible and well-balanced.

6. Support groups for dieters include:

Overeaters Anonymous, operating much like Alcoholics Anonymous and preserving the anonymity of those they help, expects members to get diet plans from their own physician. They do offer three eating plans and advice about eating, such as:
- Three moderate meals a day, with nothing between meals except low-calorie beverages.
- Avoidance of all personal binge foods.

TOPS (Take Off Pounds Sensibly), which has worked closely with the medical profession, puts emphasis upon group support. They also insist upon medical supervision of each member's diet. Dues and contributions go toward research in obesity and metabolism.

9

Which Body Type Are You?

You have a body type—we all do.

Dr. William B. Sheldon and his associates at Columbia University made a study of human physique. They classified the human body into three major types with several subtypes.

Most of us are a combination, but tend more toward one type than the others.

1. The Ectomorph

Are you the skinny type who eats constantly but never puts on weight? If so, call yourself an ectomorph.

Ectomorphs have stringy muscles, relatively narrow chests, and a shorter trunk in relation to arms and legs.

If you're an ectomorph, you probably did your best in such sports as track and tennis—which require little support of the body weight.

2. The Mesomorph

Maybe you're a mesomorph. If so, you probably played in vigorous sports that required a lot of movement. For men, that's usually football.

ECTOMORPH

MESOMORPH

ENDOMORPH

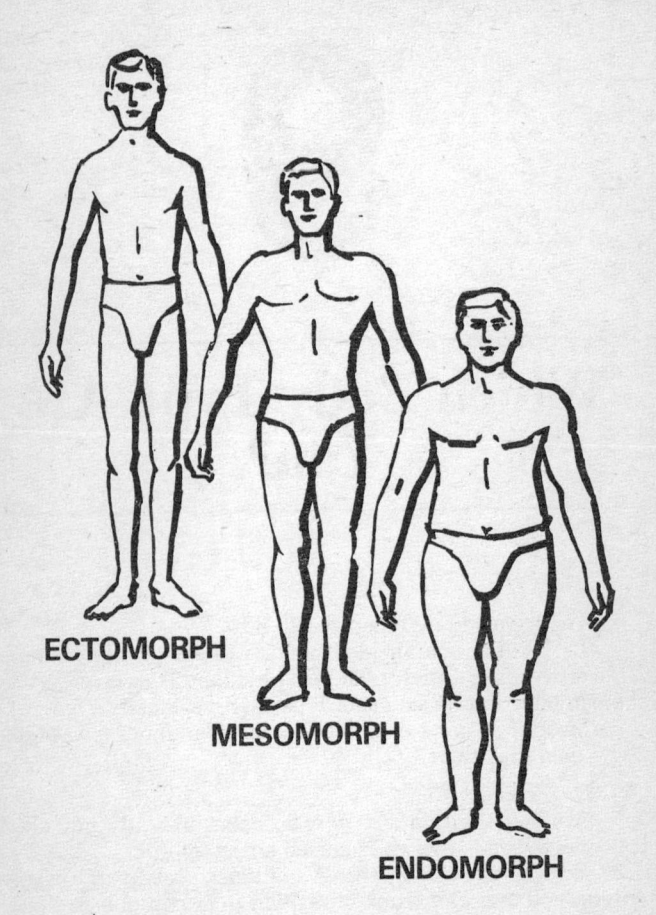

Knowing our body type tells us something about our possibilities and limitations.

Which Body Type Are You?

If you're a male, you have a solid, muscular build with broad shoulders, a massive chest, slender waist, broad hips, and large thighs.

If you're a female mesomorph, you have a solid build with firm muscles. (Women's muscles aren't ever as pronounced as men's because of the fat-tissue covering, which is greater in women of all body types.)

3. *The Endomorph*

Perhaps this fits you—you've struggled all your life with a weight problem. You have a predominance of fat tissue (although you are not necessarily obese), with a large body.

Your weight settles in the middle of your body and might even give you a pear shape.

One wise person said:

> "The prime requisite for obesity is a moderate endomorph body type without discipline."

Not sure of your body type?

Perhaps you're a *medial*. That means your body has no predominant physical features. You're of medium build and medium muscle structure.

If you're a medial, you're probably active, ambitious, and energetic. In later years, you might develop a paunch but stay lean in other areas.

Another subtype is the *ecto-medial*.

If you're the thin, wiry type with a sharp muscular shape, full of energy, fast moving, and hate to sit down, this is your body type. If you're an ecto-medial, you tend to talk fast and worry often.

How do I determine my body type?

I've listed only the major classifications, and you may not fit exactly under any one of them. But you can determine which one you *most* resemble.

Here's how:

1. Read the descriptions of the body types.
2. Compare them with yourself in a mirror. Ask, "What are my *predominant* characteristics?" (If you're still not sure, ask your mate or a friend.)
3. As you compare your own body lines with the characteristics described—regardless of height—classify yourself as the type you come closest to fitting.
4. If you have no predominant feature, classify yourself as a medial.

So what?

Jim is my jogging partner. Today, while running, I talked about body types, and we discussed whether he was a medial or a mesomorph.

Finally he asked, "So what?"

Others may ask the same question. In what particular way does it help us to know our body type?

First, it tells us something about both our limitations and possibilities.

TV commercials
> ads in newspapers and magazines
>> movies
>>> diet books and programs all scream at us
>>>> (or at least imply)

that there is an *ideal* physical form.

Even more, they imply that anyone can achieve it. But that's not possible!

I ought to know—I learned the hard way.

When I was in the seventh grade, Dwayne moved into our neighborhood, and we had many classes together. Dwayne, a classic mesomorph (even though I didn't know the term then), excelled in sports. He had, as I remember, a gigantic chest and muscular arms. He worked out with weights, and for three months I tried the same exercises because I wanted rippling muscles like Dwayne.

Nothing happened except that I wore myself out. I classify myself as an ecto-medial. No matter how hard I try, I'll never have an expansive chest or bulging biceps.

But in seventh grade I didn't know that. For months after giving up my weight lifting, I had the feeling deep inside that if only I had persisted, I might have boasted of twenty-two-inch biceps, just as Dwayne did.

Second, you can minimize undesirable physical characteristics. Being aware of my own tendency toward pushing myself and not relaxing enough, I've learned to be on guard. I've learned to rest when I need it.

Third, you can change. Anyone who follows a sensible and well-rounded fitness plan can change—sometimes radically.

This includes:

- decreasing measurements (or increasing if that is what you want)
- improving posture
- losing weight
- even correcting physical disorders.

Which Body Type Are You?

My friend Ralph fought high blood pressure most of his adult life. When he reached thirty-two, his doctor put him on a mild medication to lower his readings. Then Ralph started on a fitness program. Six months later he was able to stop taking medication, and his blood pressure reads 120/75—a good level.

Even though I had two trips to the hospital with ulcers before my fitness program, I have not had any flare-ups since starting my shape-up regimen.

Fourth, you realize that you inherit your basic body build. This inherited build includes such things as the length and thickness of muscle fibers.

Endomorphs and mesomorphs (the stocky types) have a larger digestive tract per unit of body volume as well as larger intestinal organs than the slimmer types.

Because of a greater capacity *and need*, endomorphs and mesomorphs tend to be heavier and have more body fat than ectomorphs.

We don't have to feel guilty if our body build is more like Nell Carter's than Loni Anderson's.

Fifth, exercise and diet *can* change your muscles as well as the amount of fatty tissue.

But . . .

only within limits.

You can never change your basic body build.

If you were born with a mesomorph figure, you'll never have that linear look of the top fashion models. But then, they'll never have the curves and strength you have!

However, the most important reason for knowing about your body type is:

Sixth, you can be your most attractive self.

Physical attraction doesn't limit itself to one body type.

Be the best you that you can be!

10

How Dense Are You?

Did you know that your weight could increase from 150 pounds to 160 and yet not affect your actual size?

Or your dress size could go from a twelve to a ten, and yet the scales still show you at the same weight?

How can that be?

The answer: *body density*.

Outward appearance (such as dress or shirt size) doesn't accurately indicate weight. We also need to consider the body density.

Low Body Density occurs when you don't use up the food energy you absorb. Instead you store it in the form of fatty deposits in your tissues. This initially increases *size*, not weight. People with low density have a tendency to be less healthy, even malnourished. Their bodies burn calories less efficiently. Fatty tissues are larger than other body tissues.

High body density occurs when you burn up more food energy than you absorb and have to use stored energy to keep you going. This converts the fatty contents of your tissues into muscles (firms your muscles). Muscle tissue is heavier than fat tissue. That means weight can rise while dimensions remain the same.

Stable body density means that you use the same amount of food energy that you absorb, and the density of your body remains the same.

Body density changes in all of us.

If, for instance, you become extremely active, you will have a high body density. You can eat larger-than-normal meals and your weight will stay the same or might even increase by as much as ten pounds, while your measurements remain the same.

When thinking about density, here's the rule:

> The higher the density,
> the fitter you are.

Fat-free tissues yield more energy and work with less strain. If you want to get the most from your food and to achieve the greatest freedom of movement, high density is your goal.

11

Isometric, Isotonic, and Those Other Strange Words

For the past decade, physical-fitness experts have tossed certain terms around for us to absorb.

Here are a few of the common ones:

Exercises characterized as *aerobic* (*aero* means air) are those that require the increased and steady use of oxygen for a significant period of time—usually at least twenty minutes. Using sufficient oxygen to meet the demands of these exercises that require endurance and stamina is thought to be beneficial to the cardiovascular system.

Examples of such rhythmic, sustained exercise are continuous running, bicycling, and swimming.

Anaerobic exercise results in bursts of energy production from short spurts of explosive activity. Rather than depending on oxygen for energy, fuel for this type of exercise is the carbohydrate glycogen stored in muscle fiber and released with the start of activity.

An example of anaerobic activity would be the game of racquetball. It is characterized by quickness rather than endurance.

Isometric exercises came into prominence a few years ago with the promise that men could double their muscle strength and bulk in six minutes a day by performing exercises that required approximately six seconds each.

These exercises involve contracting a muscle and holding it in a static position for a few seconds.

Example: Press your arm against a wall. The muscle is contracting, but it isn't going anywhere.

Isometrics work. Those using the exercise do build bigger, stronger muscles. *But* the muscles work best only in the position in which the exercise is being performed. That is, if you press against a wall with your arms for ten seconds a day, your muscle will become much stronger—but mostly when it performs an action similar to that of pushing against the wall. It does gain some strength throughout its entire range of motion.

Isokinetic exercises are performed on machines that provide constant resistance against the muscles as they go through the whole range of motion. The Nautilus is the best known isokinetic machine; it promises to produce greatly increased strength in a short period of time.

The disadvantage is that you need machines that are expensive and very large. You will probably have to join a health club to get the use of them.

Isotonic exercises are those in which you raise or lower a weight through the range of motion of a muscle. Most of life's activities are done with isotonic muscular contractions. Every time you pick up a box of cereal, you are doing an isotonic movement because your muscles are moving the weight of your body.

The best examples of isotonic exercises are calisthenics and weight lifting. Calisthenics includes such exercises as pull-ups and sit-ups, in which the weight of your body acts as a resistance to your muscles.

12

Toes in the Water

The first time my Dad took me swimming, I was six. My older brother and one of my sisters dashed into the water and paddled around, laughing and enjoying themselves.

I wanted to get into the water, too. But I didn't know how. I remember standing on the riverbank, sticking my toes in the cool water. My sister kept calling, "Come on in!"

"I'm scared," I called back, but I did put both feet in the water. Then I took a few steps until my knees were submerged. Each step I took was harder than the one before.

Without my expecting it, Dad came from behind, grabbed me, dunked me, and then after I paddled wildly for a few seconds, pulled me back out. He didn't let me flounder alone.

"Get back into the water and start paddling, or you'll never learn," he said.

I was afraid to try. But I didn't want another dunking. I got back into the water and inched away from him.

My brother grabbed an arm, and I had my first swimming lesson. I felt awkward and paddled stiffly, but I got into the water.

That's how exercise works, too. Just sticking a toe in the water isn't enough. You have to take a plunge and commit yourself if you're going to get into shape.

Plunging in doesn't mean setting up a three-hour daily routine. It does mean a commitment to physical fitness *and* jumping in by actually doing it!

So now you're *committed.*
    You're psyched up.
        How do you get
           from sticking in your toe
              to taking a deep plunge?

1. Be sure you're convinced of the value of and need for physical fitness.

    We find time to do anything we want. When we know shaping up is important for ourselves, then we're ready to jump in.

2. Remind yourself that even though you sweat, grunt, and it tires you the first few times, you're going to feel better about yourself after you've established the habit of physical fitness.

    Ask former flabbies. Let them tell you how much better they feel about themselves and about life. This matter of physical fitness reaches into all areas of life. For example, more than one psychiatrist now realizes that a crucial step in rehabilitation for psychiatric patients involves their seeing themselves as effective human beings. These doctors have put their patients on a physical fitness program and have noted that they learn to feel good about their bodies and about themselves.

3. Enjoy your exercise program.

    You won't stick with any program unless you enjoy it. In devising your own fitness program, make it as much fun as possible. Especially incorporate "cheating" exercises (*see* chapter 17). And give yourself at least a three-month trial to make it a vital part of your life.

4. Get positive reinforcement.

    Ask for reinforcement if you have to. Tell two or three cheerful types (avoid the pessimists) that you plan to get into shape. Explain your need for encouragement. Ask them to tell you every time they see any improvement in your appearance or attitude.

5. Begin today.

    Don't wait for a better time. (There never is a better time.) Don't wait until you can join a health club. You can do most exercises in normal clothing, any place. Schedule exercises into your daily pattern. If you can't find twenty minutes at a single period, break it up: Five minutes in the morning, five at noon, and another five before or after the evening meal. That's fifteen minutes squeezed into your day.

6. Encourage yourself.

Each day as you start your exercises, encourage yourself by saying aloud such statements as:

> "I will stick to my program."
> "I'm going to be a better me."
> "I'm going to become physically fit."

Most of us believe what we hear repeated frequently. Say your own words of self-encouragement, speaking positively of your goals and determination. You'll learn to believe that voice!

13

Before You Do Your First Exercise

Choose a time based on personal preference and daily schedule—one that you can keep *regularly*.

Regular activity is more beneficial—and healthy—than sporadic work. A four-hour Saturday session is too harsh on your system, and one day a week doesn't do enough. Plan some form of exercise for a minimum of three times a week.

Have a set schedule of exercises for yourself. (You may vary or change them later.)

Forming the habit of same-time-same-place-same-activity helps assure you of continuing with your exercise program. Don't rush. Relax when you exercise. This is time set aside just for you.

Learn to breathe properly in doing exercises.

Exhale through your mouth with lips half-closed; inhale through your nose, nostrils wide open. If you need additional air, open the windows.

Choose exercises that involve all parts of the body, separately as well as together.

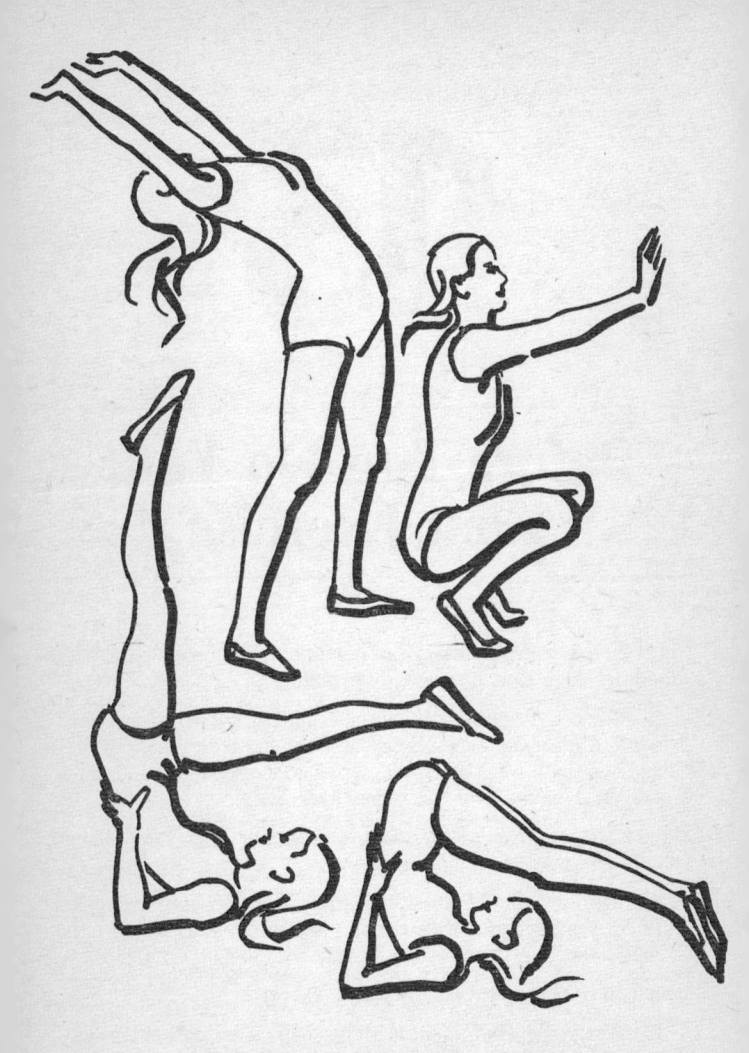

Start your exercise program by planning a set schedule of exercises for yourself.

Before You Do Your First Exercise

Don't be too ambitious.

Proceed carefully and slowly. Don't overtax yourself, especially in the beginning. Begin by performing a small number of exercises in a minimum number of repetitions. Increase this gradually but never to the point of fatigue. Moderation is your key to successful exercise and fitness.

Exercises become easier with practice.

It takes time and patience to learn new skills (remember when you learned how to drive?). Exercising becomes easier as you practice. Once you begin an exercise program and stay with it, it becomes increasingly easier.

Make at least a three-month commitment to yourself.

It often takes three months for people to establish the habit. (In running, we say it takes up to three months until people become addicted!) If you persist, exercise will become a natural part of your life. You'll find it one of the highlights of your day.

Look your best when exercising.

Sound strange? A valuable secret of successful exercise involves looking as attractive as possible at all times. The way you dress improves what you see in the mirror. Wear leotards or practice shorts that look good on *you*.

Even if you have flabby curves, you want to keep reminding yourself that they'll go away in time. Say aloud, "I'm going to be a happier, more attractive me."

Your workout clothes will help!

Do your exercises smoothly and rhythmically.

Each motion in an exercise can be learned and performed in a graceful and efficient way, without strain and without using excessive energy. Make certain you carefully follow instructions on all exercises. Follow the rhythm indicated, not in jerky motions, but in a smooth flowing count. Keep your toes pointed in the direction of the movement, hands and arms graceful. Keep your face pleasant and avoid a tense look or a grimace or labored breathing and puffing. If you have to puff to do an exercise, you are working too hard!

Plan your program carefully.

Many factors go into determining how much exercise you need. Experts base programs on your calendar age and your physical age, as well as the length of time since you last engaged in vigorous physical activity.

Calendar age is important but physical age more so. You can be old at thirty, still young at sixty—it depends on your health, your attitude, and your fitness.

If you have any question about physical exercise, talk to your doctor first.

If you're taking any regular medication, don't even put your toe into the water until you've been assured that it's okay.

And finally . . .

Don't strain.
Don't overdo—especially in the beginning.
When you get tired, *stop*.

14

A Word About Breathing

Don't hold your breath during exercise.

Holding your breath causes muscle contraction that closes the glottis (opening between the vocal cords in the larynx) which increases the pressure inside the chest cage. This action decreases the amount of blood returning to the heart, resulting in a loss of oxygen when most needed.

Improper breathing can also cause tightness in the neck, dizziness, and headaches.

Breathing freely is better for anyone—but especially for those with lung or heart disease.

For example:

In push-ups, exhale during the pushing up, inhale while lowering your body.

When running, exhale every other time your right foot strikes the ground.

During heavy exercise, if your breathing rate *exceeds* fifteen times in fifteen seconds, this is a signal to
        slow down   or   decrease the exercise.

15

Shape-Up Exercises

How do I shape up?
How do I maintain physical fitness without large amounts of time and heavy energy drain?

This chapter describes conventional exercises that affect every part of the body. Do them regularly. Once you've mastered them, you may want to add, change, or even modify them to fit your individual needs.

Time: At least fifteen minutes, three times a week. Twenty minutes daily is ideal.

Place: Anywhere you're comfortable, but as much as possible, make it the same place each time. (We're all creatures of habit and most of us are sensitive to our surroundings.)

> Be sure to incorporate suggestions
> from chapter 17 on cheating exercises.

WARM-UP EXERCISES

1. Jumping Jack. Stand with arms at side. Jump. Spread the feet to the side, and simultaneously swing the arms overhead on count of one. Then swing the arms down and jump back to the starting position on count of two. Try to do it rhythmically and at a moderate cadence.

For beginners, no more than fifteen repetitions.

2. *Deep breathing.* Stand with feet comfortably apart. Slowly swing your arms forward and upward, raise up on the toes, and inhale deeply until the arms are in an overhead position. Swing the arms down, drop to the heels, and exhale as the arms are returned to the starting position.

Repeat five times.

3. *Side Twister.* Stand with feet comfortably apart, arms extended out to the sides, palms down. Slowly twist to the side as far as you can, bob gently once, and repeat to the other side. To relieve strain on the knees, turn the far foot slightly in as you twist.

Do five on each side.

4. *Knee Bends.* Men, stand with feet comfortably apart; women, with legs together, hands on hips. Bend the legs to just short of a ninety degree angle, extending the arms forward for balance as you go down, then return and repeat in a slow to moderate cadence.

Do this ten times.

5. *Slow Jog.* Stand in place with the arms in a running position. Slowly jog in place or in a small circle for fifty counts (count only as your left foot strikes the ground).

6. *Waist Stretch.* Stand with your legs apart, arms at shoulder level, elbows bent. Twist your body to the right, keeping your hips immobile. Twist your body to the left, exhale as you twist, inhale as you straighten up.

Repeat six times.

7. *Waist and Back Balance.* Sit on the floor with your knees bent, feet off the floor, arms forward. Slowly extend one leg and then bend it. Extend the other leg, bend it, and continue for ten times, alternating legs.

8. *Hip Bump.* (For women only.) Sit on the floor, legs extended in front, lean back, arms at an angle, the weight on your palms. Lift your hips and twist your body to the left, then bump your hips on the floor. Lift hips again, twist your body to the right, and bump the floor again.

Repeat twenty-five times each side.

Shape-Up Exercises

TOP-TO-BOTTOM EXERCISES

1. *Toe Touch.* In each of the following four positions, bend down and touch the toes and then return to your starting position.
a. With feet apart at shoulder width
b. With feet together
c. With legs crossed at the knees—first with right over left
d. And then with left over right
   Repeat four times in each position.

2. *Sprinter's Drive.* Place hands on the floor at shoulder width and lean forward with your right leg well up under the chest, with the left fully extended to the rear. Alternate leg positions in a two-count rhythm as follows: (a) shift positions (b) return to the starting position.
   Do this ten times.

3. *Push-Ups.* Women, keep the knees in contact with the floor throughout the movement. Lie flat on the floor with hands directly under the shoulder joints, fingers pointing staight ahead. Straighten the arms and raise the body in a straight line from head to heels for men (from head to knees for women) to a fully extended position supported by the arms and toes (knees for women). Lower the body in a straight line by bending the arms until the chest comes to within an inch of the floor.
   Repeat in a moderate rhythm up to ten times.

4. *Sitting Stretch.* Sit with feet together, hands at the sides. Without bending the legs, bend the trunk forward, tuck the head in, reach forward as far as possible, and grasp firmly around the legs, ankles, or feet, according to the extent of your reach. Hold for the count of six, relax, and return to the starting position.
   Do five times.

5. *Side Leg Lifts.* Lie on one side with the legs together, the head supported by the elbow and hand, and the other hand on the floor in front of the body for balance. With the leg straight, lift it as far as possible and return to the starting position.
   Do ten on each side.

These basic exercises help shape up all parts of your body.

1. Master all of the exercises.
2. Do them regularly—at least twice a week.
3. Then eliminate or add exercises.

You can do them all.

    You have only 8 warm-up exercises
                +
              5 top-to-bottom exercises

            13 separate exercises

Best of all, you can do them all in about fifteen minutes!

After you've mastered these exercises and want to try a few new ones, consult books on the suggested reading list on page 94.

If any of the exercises seem difficult at first, perform only a part of it, such as a slight knee bend instead of a full bend, *but* progress until you can eventually do the full exercise.

After you can do all the exercises the suggested number of times without undue fatigue, increase the repetitions slowly by one or two a week.

16

Don't-Just-Sit-There Exercises

Even if you're sitting all day at a desk, or too tired to move from your easy chair in the evening, *you can exercise.*

And you can exercise while you're sitting!

1. Sit at edge of chair, arms crossed, feet flat on floor. Lean back slowly. Stop just before your upper back touches chair back and hold. Slowly return to sitting position. Repeat four times.
2. Sit at edge of chair, back resting against chair back, knees together and feet flat. Keeping legs tightly together and with knees bent, slowly lift legs as high as you can, keeping your back against chair back. Hold, lower, and repeat.
3. Stretch arms up to ceiling as high as you can and hold. Then stretch arms out to side, fingers pointed upward, and push out as hard as you can and hold.
4. Sitting with feet flat on floor, arms raised, and chin tucked to chest, slowly lean forward as far as you can, trying to touch forehead to knees. Slowly curl back up and repeat.
5. Sitting straight with legs stretched out, lift one leg up to at

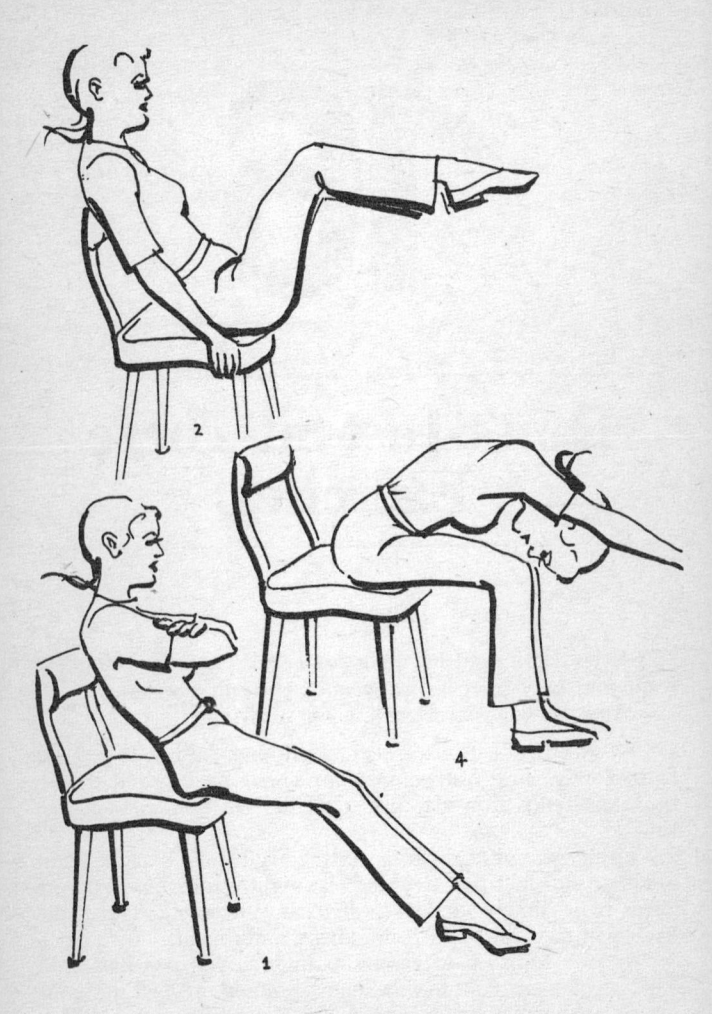

Some exercises can be done even while sitting at your desk.

Don't-Just-Sit-There Exercises

least seat level. Keeping leg lifted, flex foot toward you as far as you can and hold. Point foot as far as you can and hold. Circle foot from ankle slowly around. Reverse directions. Then circle entire leg from hip, toe pointed. Reverse directions. Repeat as many times as you can with each leg.

6. Sit straight in chair, legs stretched out, feet flexed. Keeping legs straight, slowly lift both legs as high as possible, but at least level with seat. While holding legs in air, spread them as wide as possible, then close slowly and open again, repeating as many times as you can.

17

Cheating Exercises

I heard one doctor say, "Calisthenics are fun. But they are of no real value unless they're done continuously and vigorously enough for at least ten minutes."

Maybe he's right.

But I hate doing calisthenics (even though I do them six days a week). For me, they're boring.

I persist with calisthenics because I need them. I like getting them finished so that I can do exercises I enjoy, especially running.

If you find calisthenics boring, don't despair. You can "cheat"! And you can do it fairly, too.

Sensible dieters long ago learned to cheat fairly by substituting artificial sweetener for sugar and skim milk for whole. They've learned other tricks, which help them in their weight-control problems yet appear not to demand sacrifice.

The same thing can happen when getting into shape. You can cheat—and cheat fairly!

BUT
    like creative dieting
        it still demands discipline
            commitment
                and a basic fitness plan.

Here's how I got into creative cheating.

It began during the first years of our marriage. I taught school in those days, and it meant a dress shirt five days a week and another on Sunday—at least six every week. Because this was before the days of permanent press, it meant those six shirts had to be ironed every week.

Shirley and I shared the ironing. When she started to press the first shirt, she timed herself. It took ten minutes plus a few seconds. I did my first one in slightly under ten minutes.

From then on, we played a game. We determined that the quality of the ironing must be as good as a ten-minute job. We would work to reduce the time.

Over the next few years we cut that time down to slightly under five minutes. We not only accomplished our task (ironing my dress shirts) but had fun doing it. *The game took the chore out of the work.*

Then, thirty pounds and four waist inches ago, I embarked on a fitness program. I didn't intend to look like Arnold Schwarzenegger or a member of the United States weight lifting team. I wanted to feel good and look fit.

I tried all the conventional exercise programs. Boring! I kept at the exercises with some degree of faithfulness. But each morning it was an I-guess-I'd-better-have-my-punishment-now attitude.

Then I remembered the game Shirley and I had played with ironing. But, instead of cutting off minutes, I decided to find ways to force exercise on myself that wouldn't look or feel like exercise.

And I did!

So have a lot of other people!

Let's look at some of them. After you've read through the list, perhaps you can think of your own creative ways to cheat fairly. Make it a game for yourself.

Cheating While Shopping

1. When you drive to a mall to shop, park your car as far away from the stores as possible. It's an exciting alternative to cruising up and down the lanes near the buildings, trying to find a spot closer to the store entrance.
2. Make extra trips back to your car. After you've made one or two purchases, instead of carrying several bags around, walk out to your car, put them in the trunk, and return to the mall.
3. When you buy groceries and push the cart out to your car,

Cheating Exercises

return the cart—not to the areas marked for that purpose, but all the way back to the store itself.

4. In the grocery store, instead of standing in front of the cereal, stand at least two feet away, forcing yourself to reach and/or bend to pick up the box you want.

5. Leave your shopping cart at the end of an aisle, go up the aisle, and as you pick up each item, return it to the cart and go on to the next item.

6. Extend your park-and-walk idea. Leave your car a full block from the cleaners. Why not walk a quarter of a mile to your dentist's office?

Inside Buildings

1. Don't ride elevators. Use the stairs. I decided that I would walk or run up steps to a maximum of six floors. If I have to visit the ninth floor, I walk my maximum and then take the elevator.

2. I go down the stairs for up to ten floors. Going down requires less energy. You might want to start initially with simply going down two flights and walking up one. Increase your floors over a course of months.

3. If you do ride the elevator, be creative. For instance, when I'm the sole passenger, I bend over and touch my toes as the elevator zooms upward. Or I do simple stretching exercises. When others ride with me, I do isometric exercises, such as leaning against the elevator wall and push, hold, relax; push, hold, relax. Sometimes I raise myself up and down on my toes or my heels. Occasionally I bend first to the left and then to right, assuming other passengers (if they pay any attention) will think my back is stiff and I'm loosening up a little.

4. Avoid escalators. Whenever possible, take the steps. If you're in a situation where you see no steps, then walk up the escalator. If you can't move ahead because of other people, do things such as turning around three or four times, as though wanting to look back where you came from. Or shift your weight from one leg to the other. How about carrying your briefcase instead of putting it on the moving steps? The two extra pounds shifted frequently from one arm to the other (even as you walk) provides a neat little exercise.

At work

1. Exercise when you talk on the phone.

   I receive lengthy calls every day. I have a long cord in my office (and a twenty-foot cord at home). As I listen, I move around, trying not to sit still during these lengthy conversations.

Try variations:
a. Do knee bends or side bends—the kind of exercises that don't distract your mind from listening attentively.
b. Grip the phone with your right hand, press hard, release, and then repeat. Change hands and start the exercise again.
c. Sit in your chair, back straight and tailbone against the back of the chair. Lift both legs until they are parallel with the seat of the chair. Then raise the right leg slowly as far as you can, return it slowly. Repeat using the left leg.
d. Sit straight and pull in your stomach muscles, hold a few seconds, release, and then repeat the process.

2. Don't buzz an extension. Instead, walk to that other department. Stand at the person's desk when you talk, instead of sitting.
3. Look for opportunities to carry small items. Offer to help co-workers move heavy objects. Don't scoot chairs, but lift and carry. Those few seconds of physical effort strengthens muscles most of us seldom use.
4. Bend to open drawers or file cabinets. When I open a file drawer, I stand far enough away that I have to bend. Bend from the waist, keeping legs straight.
5. Lunch breaks. If you brown bag it, go for a walk while eating, if necessary, or at least immediately afterward. Plan for at least five minutes of continuous movement before returning to work. Your afternoon will go better, and you'll have more energy.
6. Wear comfortable shoes. One way to keep moving is to wear shoes that don't make you miserable when you walk. Buy shoes that give you ease of movement and don't make your calves ache after being on them for fifteen minutes.
7. Take an exercise break every hour.

Prolonged sitting weakens muscles in the legs and can interfere with circulation. At least once an hour, *move*. Stand up and stretch. Walk down the hall for a drink of water. Open a window or close one.

8. Don't ask for anything to be brought to you. Get it yourself. People not only appreciate your coming for files or objects, but you get the added benefit of another opportunity to exercise.
9. When talking in a group, stand when you speak, or pace the room.

Cheating Exercises

At Home

1. Plan a minimum of five minutes of exercise. As soon as you get home from work, shopping, dinner, or merely visiting the neighbors, take five minutes for physical activity. Play with the cat. Crawl with the baby, on your hands and knees. Put on a record and waltz or skip around the room. Put the dog on a leash and walk the animal for at least five minutes.

2. If you have more than one level in your house or apartment, keep your coat or purse on a different level from the front door. If you're on a single level, keep the purse or coat in a room as far from the door as possible, giving you the excuse to move that much more.

3. Get dressed creatively. Exaggerate your motions. Bend over to put on a shoe (never sit), or balance yourself on one foot as you put the shoe on the other. When putting on a shirt or blouse over your head, stretch. Stand on your tiptoes as you comb your hair.

4. Walk across the room, taking ten steps holding your abdomen in. Relax. Do it a second time.

5. When you leave the house and go to the car or the mailbox, hold in your abdominal muscles. Find ways to do this on short walks you do regularly, and it'll soon become a habit.

6. In the kitchen, it may take longer to prepare meals, but you can cheat by making every motion separate. Don't keep the salt at the back of the stovetop. Place it far enough away that you have to twist your body to reach it and twist a second time to return it. When setting the table, don't grab plates, glasses, and silverware at one time. Make the plates a trip, return for the glasses, and then the silverware.

7. In the bathroom:

    a. When brushing your teeth, jiggle to the count of fifteen as you brush your uppers. Then fifteen as you brush your lowers.

    b. As you comb your hair, jiggle up and down. Swing your hips. Play the radio or sing, and move your body in time to the music.

    c. Keep your cosmetics far enough away from the sink that you force yourself to reach for them. Stretch as far as you can for the deodorant or other items.

    d. When you finish with your facecloth, twist it as hard as you can, wringing out the water. Hold that tension a few seconds. Then twist it as hard as you can in the opposite direction.

    e. Hold the cloth against your chest and then, pulling

with both arms, you stretch an entirely different set of muscles than those mentioned above.

    f. Do knee bends in the shower.

    g. When you dry off, lift your legs high, bend forward when you towel off your back. Stretch upward and even stand on your tiptoes when you dry off your arms.

8. Make the laundry a fun thing.

At our home I do the laundry every week. First I carry the clothes hamper down the steps and dump all the clothes on the floor. Then I pick up each item separately and put it in its proper pile. This causes me to bend a lot. When loading the machine, I pick up each piece, one at a time, place it in the washer, then bend down to pick up the next.

9. Try it with dishwashing. If you use an automatic washer or do your dishes in the sink, discover ways to bend, stretch, or move. One woman told me that she does a simple kind of soft-shoe dance at the sink.

10. Avoid time-saving and effort-saving gadgets.

You don't need to go back to the hand lawnmower (although that's great exercise!), but don't use push buttons for opening garage doors. Instead, think of the great opportunity to reach down, pull up the garage door (which means lifting a heavy object), and then later closing it by pulling it all the way to the floor again.

Don't use remote control for television. This gadget only encourages you to sit longer. When you do change channels, jump up! If you're not too embarrassed with others around (or you're alone), why not get on your hands and knees and crawl to the set, change channels, and crawl back?

11. Commercial breaks during TV time can be more than moving to and from the refrigerator. Instead, make each break (or at least each half hour) an opportunity for exercise.

    a. Jog in place. March in place.

    b. Do knee bends.

    c. Place a broom handle (or any long stick) across your shoulders, with your arms grasping either end. Stand straight, bend to the right, without moving your hips or legs. Then to the left.

    d. If you have a stationary bicycle, do your pedaling then.

    e. Stand straight, then lean over and place your hands on the back of the sofa, and swing your waist and hips.

    f. Jump rope.

Cheating Exercises

Now it's your turn:
> Follow these cheating exercises.
>> Discover your own ways to cheat fairly.

Some bright person set up three rules for attaining physical fitness:
1. Don't lie down when you can sit.
   2. Don't sit when you can stand.
      3. Don't stand when you can move.

18

Stick With It

If you're like most people, you'll want to give up your exercise program after one or two weeks. That's the time to say, "I'm going to stick with it."

The most common reason for giving up? *Boredom.*

The first few times it probably will be boring—from the time you learn the routine until you've made exercise a firmly ingrained habit. You become aware of the effort and repetition involved, and your brain might interpret all that as boredom. It may also be in your attitude. If you expect it to be dreary, you'll probably find it so. However, trying to psych yourself up by saying, "I'll enjoy every minute of it," won't work either.

If you can keep in mind the *purpose* of your shape-up program, you'll be able to stick with it. You're working to improve your overall appearance, to enhance your health, not merely to fill in ten minutes a day with activity.

Here's good news, though: The longer you work out regularly, and the longer you continue to exercise, the less you're aware of boredom. As physical exercise becomes a part of your life, your body actually looks forward to doing it—you become addicted.

You also get better at the exercises, and that increases your sense of accomplishment. Your muscles start to feel good and exercise seems natural.

But . . .

how long does it take for exercise programs to begin to feel good?

It varies from person to person. I always urge people to stick with a program for three months. By then they're hooked.

But, until your exercise has become a firmly ingrained habit, you'll probably have to exert extra willpower to do your workouts.

If you find yourself avoiding the exercise program, ask yourself *why*. Is it boredom? That will go away. Pain? Pain from exertion is transitory and slight—some people even find this kind of pain pleasurable. Examine your reasons—and then do your shape-up anyway.

Yet even after exercise has become firmly established, you'll find days when you won't feel like exercising or when exercise sessions will be unpleasant.

Most people who work out regularly have down days. To help get you past that, I have a few suggestions.

1. Distract yourself. Work out to music. When I run, I find memorization helpful—Bible verses or poetry. A few years ago, my wife and I ran with small, homemade cards that fit into our palms—she studied Spanish, and I worked on Greek.
2. Listen to the radio—especially an all-news station. You can buy transistor radios you can carry on your body while you shape up.
3. Vary your routine of exercises. Change the place you work out for a few days.
4. Keep a record. Jot down your daily workout, including the exercises, the number of repetitions, and time spent. When I first started doing calisthenics, this kept me going—because I had to give account to myself. Some prefer a loose-leaf notebook with details noted of how they felt, alongside information on daily weight and body measurements. Whatever log or journal you decide on, keep it faithfully.
5. Trick yourself. When I've started to work out and don't feel like completing my exercises, I say to myself, "I'll only do one-third of them today," to get myself started, allowing myself to quit if I need to. Usually, however, once I get into the motion of exercise, I find I can keep going.

Stick With It

6. Remind yourself constantly of the positive results of shaping up.

> "I'll look better."
> "I'll age slower" (which we know is true).
> "I'll fit into my clothes better."
> "I'll have more strength . . . more energy."

7. After you've exercised, remind yourself of how good you feel. Most people have a great sense of well-being afterward.

8. If all else fails, plan to write a book on the subject. Then you'll have to shape up—*and stay in shape!*

19

To Sleep ...

Sleep is like food: Everyone has different needs. Factors such as heredity, age, health, personality, and life-style dictate the amount of sleep you need.

Generally, everyone can fit into one of two categories.

1. Short sleepers. These folks tend to be dynamic, action oriented, energetic, ambitious, eager to excel. They waste little time worrying, and when problems hit, they lose themselves in their work. Many successful business people, career soldiers, and politicians fit into the short-sleepers category.

2. Long sleepers. These individuals (anyone who needs more than eight and one-half hours) are apt to be artists, philosophers, writers—people who use the sleep to work out new ideas in their minds. They're also apt to worry more.

HINTS FOR BETTER SLEEP

1. Try to get to sleep at the same time every night. Stick to a schedule as much as possible.
2. Make sure that the hours you sleep are the right ones for you. Keep a sleep log. Evaluate your time of going to bed, aris-

ing, amount of sleep. Over a period of months, you can see a helpful pattern for yourself.

3. Try napping during the day. Ten to twenty minutes is enough. Even if you only lie down and just relax, it's almost as good as sleep.

4. Exercise—but not just before bed. Most bodies need two hours after vigorous exercise to slow down again.

5. Don't work on important matters before going to bed. Let your brain slow down.

6. Avoid sleeping pills. A set routine can set up patterns that bring about sleep just as well as pills. Habits are also cheaper, with no side effects.

7. Relax before going to bed.

8. Don't go to bed hungry. A drop in blood sugar during the night can interfere with your sleep. Snack *lightly* on high protein foods such as milk, cheese, eggs—all rich in amino acids, which are converted by the body into serotonin, a chemical in the brain that induces sleep naturally.

9. Sleep in a comfortable bed.

10. Keep cool. Many sleep in conditions that are too warm. Studies indicate that we sleep best at a temperature just under seventy degrees.

11. Have sex, but only if it relaxes you. If you find yourself invigorated, have sex in the morning.

20

An Added Bonus: Sharper Minds!

Doctors at San Diego State University tested the reaction times of sixty-four men and women, ages twenty-three to fifty-nine. Half were runners, the others were sedentary. The test measured how fast each participant could react to either of two lights by releasing either the right or left index finger from a switch.

Results: The nonexercisers showed a gradual increase in reaction time, coinciding with their increase in age.

Runners, however, showed no lengthened reaction time! The oldsters proved every bit as quick as the youngsters.

Conclusion: Exercise seems to force the same kind of adaptations on brain cells as it does on muscles. It has to do with enzyme activity and blood flow.

If reaction time seems a crude measure of mental aging, the researchers argued, "It provides an excellent indication of how effectively and efficiently the processes of the central nervous system are working." They also use the same device to measure degrees of senility.

21

Results?

While medical research has made giant strides in the past few years, its contribution to American health is shared with an increased awareness of physical fitness by Americans.

Americans *are* getting into shape.

Look at these statistics:

> Heart disease, American's number-one killer, has decreased 20 percent since 1967.

Strokes have dropped more than 30 percent during the same period.

> > Life expectancy in the United States has now risen to a record seventy-three years.

> Because of increased awareness of the cholesterol controversy, we Americans now eat eight pounds less beef per person in a year than we did in 1970.

Smoking among the young is declining
> (especially among females) and
> > 1.8 million smokers kicked the habit between 1978 and 1980.

Most states now prohibit smoking in elevators.
> Hospitals post restricted areas for smoking.
> > Smart restaurateurs offer a nonsmoking section.

Remember when President John F. Kennedy expressed his concern over the lack of fitness in our nation? In 1960, he said,

"Our growing softness,
  our increasing lack of physical fitness,
    is a menace to our security."

In the generation since, we have reversed the situation.
  We are a nation getting into shape!

22

Miscellaneous Fitness Tips

1. Exercise alone isn't enough for fitness. When you combine a physical regimen with healthy dietary habits, you can then expect to get in shape—and stay there. Someone said, "Exercising without obeying the rules of health is like swallowing two pills—the first makes you feel great, the second counteracts it."
2. The slogan of the American Health Foundation is: Die young as late as possible! Keeping physically fit helps make that slogan a reality.
3. Before you get into an exercise program, especially if you have been inactive for a long time, *start slowly*. Don't overdo—especially in the beginning.
4. The best time to exercise: regularly. Whatever time of day you prefer, aim for a schedule that keeps you exercising at least three times a week.
5. A set schedule is the easiest way to be faithful to a fitness program. Know when you will exercise and for how long. Don't rush into your exercises.
6. Breathing: Exhale through your mouth, lips half-closed, in-

hale through your nose, nostrils remaining wide open. If indoors, you may also want to open windows for additional air.

7. Begin by performing a few repetitions. Increase this number gradually, but never to the point of fatigue. Moderation leads to successful exercise as well as fitness.

8. Sleep: The amount you need depends on your age, habits, and needs. Some require only four or five hours; others as many as nine. The most restful (or deep) sleep usually occurs just after the first hour of slumber and then slowly lessens until you awaken.

9. Try napping! If you can take a ten-to-twenty-minute rest, you can recharge your batteries and start out fresh again.

10. Stick with it! You'll probably be tempted to quit after the first week or two. Commit yourself to stay with your fitness program for *at least three months*.

11. If you lack the personal discipline to set up your program and stick with it, then consider (a) recruiting one or two others to get into shape with you or (b) joining a health spa or community center that offers physical exercise.

23

If You've Got the Money...

Have you thought about a fitness vacation?
> Thousands have—
>> and actually go!

Health resorts have sprung up across the United States in the past decade. Originally labeled "fat farms" and limited only to the very rich, these spas are now reaching toward those in the more moderate income bracket.

Dedicated to helping people lead a healthier life-style, they cater to those who can scarcely walk across the room without puffing, as well as to those who are already trim—and want to stay that way.

There are luxury programs in posh settings and others aimed at more economical fitness. They help clients break bad eating habits, begin healthier diets, get started on exercise programs, and move toward a greater sense of well-being.

Figures indicate that approximately 200 permanent health-resort facilities exist in the United States, of which only 25 percent existed before 1970. These figures don't include programs run by doctors, clinics, and hospitals.

Prices vary at these health resorts. Figures (1982) go from under $500 a week for a quality program of nutrition and exercise to as much as $2500 a week. Some resorts offer weekend specials for $150 to $350.

Most of these have grown out of the holistic health movement and are a far cry from summer programs and camps for overweight youngsters. Seventh-Day Adventists, pioneers in nutrition among Christian groups, run such facilities throughout the United States. Most of their programs last a month, beginning with a physical examination, and include exercise programs, and a dietary program with vegetarian meals. They feature lectures and seminars on spiritual and mental well-being and health.

Although this may be out of the price range for many, one couple said. "It was the only way we could get started. Once we had help in knowing *how* to start, we've been able to maintain a program of fitness through exercise and diet."

... Maybe it's not so expensive, after all!

24

Finally . . .

At the beginning of this book I explained how I got into physical fitness. After nearly a decade, I'm more committed to keeping my body in shape than ever before.

I'm not trying to win any prizes. I'll never look like a professional athlete. I exercise regularly and stay in shape for myself.

And for God.

Perhaps those last three words sound strange, but

God made my body and I'm responsible for caring for it.

For Further Reading

Clark, Linda. *Know Your Nutrition.* New Canaan, Conn.: Keats Publishing, Inc., 1973. This impressive paperback tells everything you'll need to know about various nutrients.

Fixx, James. *The Complete Book of Running.* New York: Random House, 1977. Of all the books on running, this is the most complete (and the best).

Jackson, Douglas W., and Pescar, Susan. *The Young Athlete's Handbook.* New York: Everest House, 1981. The subtitle, "A Guide to Sports Medicine and Sports Psychology for Parents, Teachers, Coaches, and Players," accurately describes the contents of this book.

Kounovsky, Nicholas. *The Joy of Feeling Fit.* New York: E. P. Dutton, 1971. Sensible exercise book using what he calls the Sixometric tests and a program for the total body.

Lakein, Alan. *How to Get Control of Your Time and Your Life.* New York: Peter W. Wyden, Inc., 1973. The oldest and the best on the subject.

Lappe, Frances Moore. *Diet for a Small Planet.* New York: Ballantine Books, Inc., 1975. Although nearly a decade old, it's the classic on high-protein, meatless eating, with much helpful information and 200 pages of recipes.

Marshall, John L., M.D., with Barbash, Heather. *The Sports Doctor's Fitness Book for Women.* New York: Delacorte Press, 1981. Helpful and well-written; probably the best book on fitness for women.

Morehouse, Laurence E., Jr., and Gross, Leonard. *Total Fitness in Thirty Minutes a Week.* New York: Simon and Schuster, Inc., 1975. Although the book has been out for several years, it has won wide recognition, and the program is widely used.

Solomon, Neil, with Harrison, Evalee. *Doctor Solomon's Proven Master Plan for Total Body Fitness and Maintenance.* New York: G.P. Putnam's Sons, 1976. Extremely readable and helpful.

"Executive Fitness Newsletter." Emmaus, Pa.: Rodale Press. This is a semimonthly, four-page newsletter on fitness, covering both diet and exercise, including the latest research information.